The Hair Loss Detective Presents

The Ultimate Guide to

Hair Loss Solutions

Volume Two

By

Leola Anifowoshe, Chief Trichologist

The Author

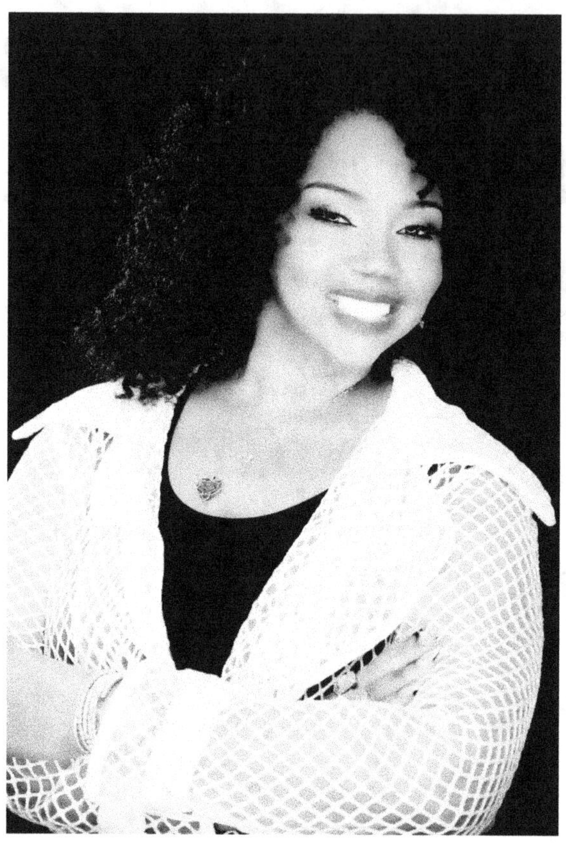

Meet, Chief Trichologist, Leola Anifowoshe, the Founder of

Solutions Hair Restoration and Wellness Center. Trichologist

Leola has been a hair restoration professional for over 25 years.

She keeps her skills modern by attending and hosting hair

shows, participating in continuing professional education, and staying closely informed about what's new and effective in the hair restoration and replacement industry.

Ms. Leola is also the Founder of Nzuri Hair Care and Wellness Products. She is passionate about what she does for her patients: how to give people their hair back in the most flattering and undetectable way is always on her mind. As an herbalist and holistic nutrition practitioner sine 1995, Trichologist Leola fully understands the causes of hair loss and offers the right Solution. She has won National awards in hair replacement and also does hair show platform work teaching other cosmetologists her special skill. She is a member of several professional organizations including the National Alopecia Foundation for People of Color, the National Cancer Awareness Committee, The Natural Hair Sorority and the Natural Hair Society.

Through years of extensive training, research and thousand of satisfied clients later, Solutions Hair Restoration has created a multi-therapeutic approach to helping people who suffer from hair loss or slow hair growth problems. "At Solutions, the only goal is to ensure that you leave with a complete solution not a quick fix," says Trichologist Anifowoshe. "When I started in hair care and wellness some 23 years ago I had no idea that my products Nzuri hair growth vitamins and natural hair services would grow to help so many people reclaim their natural born hair back by utilizing our specialized products.

Anifowoshe, Leola

Hair Loss Solutions Volume Two/ by Leola Anifowhoshe

Solutions Hair Restoration Publications

Dedication

This book is dedicated to my family that has been with me through my entire journey and to my clients that mean the world to me.

Foreword

I am sincerely honored for the invitation to write the Foreword to this absolutely eye-opening book about the mysteries of hair growth and hair loss. What is more, it is not only a source of great pleasure, but also one of total personal gratification to have the privilege of endorsing the work of someone I consider an exceptional person. That is why, in feeling uncommonly blessed to have the rare privilege of celebrating the work of the author, a valued and respected associate of mine, I also consider it an honor to comment on her written work.

The author Leola is a pacesetter, and an entrepreneurial icon in the American Hair Care industry. Those who preach that in every adversity is the seed of an equal and greater benefit may have had this remarkable lady in mind. Although she had developed her awareness of a prodigious interest in beauty, vitamins, health, and wellness quite early in life, it was her later battle with Sarcoidosis that brought her into invaluable knowledge of the overall significance of alternative medicine and nutritional supplements. The rest of her story is simply an incredible story of professionalism and entrepreneurship, as today, she is an acclaimed Master Herbalist, Holistic Therapist and Consultant Trichologist, with eminent specialization in hair loss and repair. In fact, her pedigree in the industry is so unimpeachable that she can be easily called a 'Hair Loss Detective,' solving the mystery of hair loss one strand at a time. Furthermore, her constant research on the physiology of the scalp, and her commitment to the community with reference to the Little Miss "Happy" Head beauty pageants ensures that young girls come into an early and properly-articulated understanding of hair care.

Is the author truly qualified to write a book such as this? My response is an unequivocal "Yes!" After creating Nzuri Elixir, her first and roaringly successful hair product, she went ahead to host her first natural hair show in Houston, Texas, in 2012. Since then, her extraordinarily successful and rapidly evolving brand has introduced in excess of one hundred products that include hair growth shampoos, conditioners and oils. In fact, in my opinion, this book could not be making its debut in a more timely season. I say this because there has never been a more appropriate time in the history of mankind that committed entrepreneurship demands first class professional acumen. It is this unique and original expertise in the art of hair restoration that qualifies the author to be able to write a book that will be of benefit to all stakeholders in the hair care industry.

As a truly alert learner, and a consummate networker and collaborator herself, the author has obviously deployed passion and creativity to hair restoration. Creativity is the active activity of creating something. Because of this, it seems there are many items one will see in the NZURI product line. We must remember that the author had to beat a retreat to the basics, by working with some of the best people in the wellness industry. This led to the creation of her own line of products for NZURI, and as the author herself admits, a compelling issue, Right from the beginning, was to ensure that her ingredients are always of the highest quality, and therefore, as a 100% African American owned and operative hair restoration company, her mission remains the provision of high quality and affordable hair care solutions.

Once more, in my opinion, a subscription to such a high degree of excellence can only lead to equally excellent results. That is why this book is so timely, and so appropriate. And that is why I sincerely commend the book to you. It is a book of simple utility in its delivery of both knowledge and solutions on the distressing subject of hair loss. Additionally, the author has not only presented her work in such a way as to make for infinitely easy reading, assimilation and application, the book is also one finished in exquisite literary taste. Happy reading.

Sam Ennon

BOBSA

President

CEO

Contents

Section One

Hope for Hair Loss

There is Hope for Your Hair Loss

Hair loss is a common problem among women. It is often one that women do not wish to discuss but by opening up on the topic and getting support could mean the difference between keeping your hair and losing it. Common reason that women don't speak up on hair loss is shame, embarrassment and feeling hopeless. However there are new resources that can help with your condition and bring you hope and inspiration.

One of the first things that you should do when facing hair loss is to educate yourself on conditions and then pull together a team that can help you to get through your loss. Get your medical doctor involved to rule out certain health issues that may impact your hair, next consider the services of a dermatologist because of their understanding of skin conditions and next connect with a trichologist because their specialty is treatment of the scalp.

Most people have not heard of a trichologist. However, their field of specialty has been around for generations.

Trichology is fairly new to the world. Although it originated in the United Kingdom in 1902 and slowly made its way across the world, it is still a rather unknown specialty. There are not yet any laws that govern trichology, therefore anyone who can read a book can call themselves a trichologist. Since there are no medical diagnosis given, or medications prescribed, it is not a crime. However, there are associations of trichologists around the world that organize to make sure that this field of study has structure and organization.

Experts advise extreme caution when selecting a trichologist. People suffering from hair loss are extremely vulnerable and there are plenty of con artist that would take advantage of the fact that they do not have to be governed. To find a good trichologist, do a simple Google search for hair salons or associations in the state that you live. Experts also advise that you ask for references of past clients and if they were happy with the results. It will make you feel much more at ease.

Develop a Strategy for Your Recovery

As you decide what is best for your path, here are some things that we would highly suggest that you consider.

What is the real reason that you are having hair loss?

Be willing to spend the time investigating so that you can conclude the best path for your hair recovery. Understand the importance of building a good relationship with your hair care team and especially your physician that can help provide the right diagnosis.

Identify the extent of your hair loss.

When you first notice your hair loss it can be very scary. But you have to go beyond your fears in order to halt the progression. The sooner that you do this, the more effective your hair treatments and recovery will be.

How far are you willing to go with your hair treatment options?

Access and begin treating the condition immediately. It is better for your recovery. Therefore you have to make a decision about how much that you are willing to spend, whether you want your approach to be natural, or natural plus medication. You may need to also consider your tolerance for trying new methodologies. In the end, unless you believe in the process and are fully committed, it will impact your level of recovery.

Are you all in?

There are no miracle potions to resolving hair care loss. It is a timely process that will require patience. You will have to be aware that there are no over night successes. This process will require that you stick with it and have faith that things are getting better. Treatments take a significant amount of time to show the recovery rate. Are you willing to stay with the program long term? Are you all in?

Understanding How Your Hair Grows

Hair grows in three states – Anagen, Catagen and Telogen. In the first stage (Anagen) a new hair is produced and this is the stage where most growth occurs. This phase is for a specific duration and is also genetically responsible for hair length. It is believed that there are about 100,000 hair follicles.

Next, in the Catagen (Regressive) stage, the hair has stopped growing but is yet to shed. In the final stage (Telogen) the hair is resting and eventually falls out, and a new one begins to grow. Hair growth is also sensitive to the seasons. Some believe that hair growth increases in the winter and diminishes in the summer.

In Pattern Baldness, DHT (Dihydrotestosterone) miniaturizes hair follicles by shortening the Anagen (growth) stage and at the same time can also lengthen the Telogen (resting) stage. This is usually a gradual process, and the end result is an increase in the number of short, thin hairs that are barely visible above the scalp.

There is hope, because while any hair is growing then various treatments can be administered to re-balance/block the DHT and promote healthier hair growth once again. There is no single hair loss treatment that works for everyone. In fact, it would be quite amazing if someone used a single baldness treatment that completely solved their problem.

How Long do the Hair Phases Last?

Anagen – Three-year cycles

Catagen – Approximately ten days

Telogen – Approximately three months

The best hair loss treatment is in fact a combination of the best-known products in a way that is tailored to your individual circumstances.

Generally, the most effective regime for preventing/reversing hair loss is a combination of 3 or 4 products:

1) DHT Inhibitors - Work to inhibit the negative effects of DHT

2) Growth Stimulators - artificially stimulate growth in the hair follicle

3) Hair vitamins - these products actually provide all the clinical proven vitamins and minerals required to help hair grow to its fullest and thickest

4) Hair and Scalp Cleaners - these products provide proper hair and scalp hygiene and nutrition.

In all cases, the most effective hair loss treatment will involve a combination of the above options. Since hairs grow at a slow rate it is best to do all that you can to preserve your hair.

Common Types of Hair Loss

Genetics, hormonal imbalance, improper hair care, health issues and diet commonly cause hair loss. Taking a closer look at these areas will often expose the root cause of your hair loss. Your goal is to begin your trail by examining which of these paths or combinations thereof seem to be more highly associated with your condition. Then get your hair team involved to properly assess the situation.

In men hormone imbalance within testosterone contributes to hair loss. High levels of DHT contribute to male baldness. Women can also experience hair loss from hormonal imbalance. The main hormone responsible is the thyroid hormone and certain anti-bodies that contribute to hair loss. If there is too little or too much thyroid activity the scalp can become affected causing rapid hair loss. Your medical provider can run tests to determine if these hormones issues are impacting your hair.

Women can also be impacted by hormone imbalance after pregnancy. Higher levels of estrogen can cause hair to grow. Most women take prenatal vitamins that can help boost growth during pregnancy also, but those gains can be lost after pregnancy due to hormonal imbalance while estrogen levels deplete.

Health conditions contribute to hair loss. These conditions may be through common conditions like infections or more serious conditions such as cancer. Chemotherapy can really be destructive on hair growth. In this condition women's hair breaks off during combing. Some woman have experience large losses of hair during this time.

Improper hair care can come from a variety of sources. They would include an unhealthy scalp due to improper hair care, extended use of relaxers, or coloring. It could also be caused by the way the hair is styled. Long term use of hair braiding can contribute to traction alopecia.

Diet plays a role in hair loss. A healthy diet helps to provide the nutrients necessary for healthy hair and hair growth. To be deficient in these areas is a major contributor to hair loss.

Stress and Hair Loss

People often fail to realize how stress affects physical health as well as hair health. However, it affects the overall health of an individual. This does not mean stress is always bad. Sometimes, stress is good for making an individual focused towards an approach and deciding better. In fact, some people perform better under stress and do much better. Stress up to a certain level is good, although there are no fixed parameters to establish up to what level it is good but sever stress leads to disease like anxiety, sudden hair loss and other physical health problems. Many of the people associate stress directly with sudden hair loss.

Telogen Effluvium is a kind of hair loss that occurs due to sever or sudden stress. Heavy stress in a person does the shedding of hair that pushes premature hair follicles into the resting phase. Sudden hair loss due to stress in a person appears within 2 to 3 months after facing of some stressful situations. Although, our hair falls daily and falling of about 100 hairs per day is considered very normal. In stressful circumstances a person loses almost 300 – 400 hair per day. Sudden hair loss is temporary in most of the cases. However, in some of the cases the sudden hair loss problem undergoes continue till the problem of stress is solved.

There is a well said quote, 'every problem has a solution', and so the problem of sudden hair loss too. Treating sudden hair loss naturally is one of the best way to solve the problem. Are you wandering, how?

Here are few tips to solve your hair loss problems and easing your level of stress:

Do physical exercises: Your body secrets out a hormone called adrenaline that is good for you but when body secrets this hormone in excess, this causes stress and sudden hair loss. Doing regular exercise and physical workout reduces the level of adrenaline hormone in your body. If you do physical workout on a regular basis, your body and mind will be relaxed and you will get much better sleep. Your health will also improve as a result of physical exercise.

Take enough sleep and relax: Take proper sleep and do some relaxation. You do not need special techniques to do relaxation. Only you need a peaceful place, which you have to create, be it your bedroom or office desk. Just sit in good posture, keep your body straighten, do some deep breathing and focus on good thoughts.

You can use your office desk during a short tea break or lunch hour to do the same. Include relaxation in your daily routine for 20 minutes or so, daily. You will notice the significant change in your lifestyle once you start doing this stress busting exercise. Good sleep is very important in easing stress. Sleep enough and sleep properly to ease your symptom of stress.

Once your level of stress or adrenaline in your body starts dipping, the hair loss will automatically decrease.

Have a good diet: Eat a good diet. Take diet rich in proteins, vitamins and minerals in sufficient amount. Eat whole grain breads, dairy products (milk, cheese, butter, etc) and poultry products like eggs and chicken. Also include in your diet fishes and meats. Avoid added sugars. Eat a lot of leafy green vegetables and whole fruits.

Doing all of the above will help you in staying in good shape and relieve your stress. This ultimately will solve your sudden hair loss problems.

Helping Your Hair From a Cellular Level - Nutrients

The use of natural vitamin supplements is good for human hair. It has been proven that due to stressful life style and lack of nutritious diets people are losing their hair in young age.

Modern diets have contributed to the bad health of people. It is seen that the food taken by people lacks in nutritional quality. Given the circumstances, intake of nutritional intake is a good idea. Natural vitamin supplements and herbal nutritional supplements are useful for general health as well as health of the hair. Many people take natural vitamin supplements to make up for the lack of nutrition in their food.

There are vitamins useful for hair as well as general health. Some vitamins useful for the hair are the following:

- Vitamin A – An antioxidant, vitamin A helps to produce healthy sebum in the scalp. People should take 5, 000 IU of intake per day. This vitamin is found in food like fish, meat, cheese, liver oil, eggs, cabbage, milk, carrots, spinach, broccoli, apricots and peaches.

- Vitamin B2 – Intestinal flora is responsible for the production of vitamin B2 in the human body. This vitamin is required by the human body for metabolism of amino acids, fatty acids and carbohydrates. It is most beneficial for the skin, hair and nails. Its deficiency may result in hair loss. Vitamin B2 should be a part of natural vitamin supplements you take.

- Vitamin B6 – The presence of vitamin B6 prevents hair loss and helps in production of melanin, the pigment which gives hair its color. Vitamin B6 is found in food such as liver, grains, cereals, vegetables, meat and egg yolk. It should be taken in the amount of 1.6 mg per day. It plays a key role in red blood cell metabolism and cellular growth. Vitamin B6 is also responsible for the production of hemoglobin, a compound within the red blood cells that carries oxygen to body tissue.

- Vitamin B3 – Vitamin B3 is more effective when it is used in combination with biotin. It has a positive effect on hair growth by reducing cholesterol, which when produced in the scalp sebaceous glands can trigger the formation of DHT.

- Vitamin C – It is a natural anti-oxidant and helps maintain healthy hair and skin. It should be taken in the amount of 60 mg per day. It is richly found in citrus fruit, kiwi, pineapple, tomato, green pepper, potato, green pepper, etc.

- Vitamin E – It is found in soybean, dried bean and green vegetables. This vitamin is helpful in hair growth as it increases scalp blood circulation. It should be taken in the amount of 400 IU daily.

With the proper use of natural vitamin supplements and herbal nutritional supplements you can improve your health that will contribute to the overall improvement in your life.

Iodine

Iodine is vital to your hair growth. Sheep farmers long ago found that vegetation-lacking iodine due to iodine-depleted soil would adversely affect the growth of wool in their sheep.

Likewise, to avoid hair loss, you need iodine. Iodine is synthetically added to table salt, however in this form it is not assimilated well into your body and can therefore cause iodine overload.

An excess of iodine in the body can adversely affect the thyroid. The lack of iodine can cause hypothyroidism. In hypothyroidism, your cell metabolism slows down and body cells and hair cells don't receive the energy they need to function properly. When you lack iodine, you will lose more hair than normal and may even lose eyebrow hair.

You can check your thyroid with a basal thermometer, not a digital thermometer, by placing it in your underarm first thing when you wake up.

Then, don't move for 10 minutes. After 10 minutes, look at the temperature. The normal body temperature for good thyroid function is 97.8 to 98.2 degrees C. Take this measurement for 5-10 day. If your temperature is below 97.6 and lower, for the 5-10 days, you will want to consult your doctor or for more direction and information. You definitely have low thyroid function.

Menstruating women should start this 5-10 day check on the 3rd day of their cycle.

It is best to use non-iodized salt and get your iodine from natural foods. These include seaweed, salmon, seafood, lima beans, molasses, eggs, potatoes with the skin on, watercress and garlic.

Silica

One of the most difficult nutrients vital to your hair growth to get in your diet is trace mineral silica. Silica is a form of silicon and is the second most abundant element in the earth's crust, second only to oxygen. The Earth provides everything we need for health, and with silicon being so abundant, it would seem that there would never be a problem with silica deficiency.

Unfortunately, trace minerals are rare in our diets because our food is processed and our soil depleted by chemical treatments.

Silica provides strength to your hair, and although it will not necessarily stop your hair from falling out from the follicle, it will stop hair breakage.

Silica works by stimulating your cell metabolism and formation, which slows the aging process. Foods that are rich in silica are rice, oats, lettuce, parsnips, asparagus, onion, strawberry, cabbage, cucumber, leek, sunflower seeds, celery, rhubarb, cauliflower, and swiss chard.

Try to buy these vegetables from organic sources. Note that many of these foods, particularly rice, are a large part of Asian diets and Asians tend to have the strongest and healthiest hair.

For best results eat all your fruits and vegetables raw. For certain vegetables that need to be cooked, steam them for only a few minutes.

Be sure to test your thyroid even though doctor's tests show you do not have a thyroid problem. The basal temperature test is sometimes more sensitive than blood tests taken by doctors. If you have hyperthyroidism, you will definitely have hair loss.

Herbal Therapy For the Hair

Herbal hair loss treatments have been proven effective for decades and in some cases even centuries. They cause no side effects, cost less than any other hair loss treatment and bring good results in preventing hair loss, stopping hair loss and regrowing hair.

Here are some of the most common herbs for hair loss:

1. Rosemary (Rosmarinus in Latin) – known for stimulating hair growth and for enhancing dark hair.

2. Dong Quai – A Traditional Chinese herb that contains phytoestrogens that reduces the formation of DHT. Hence, Dong Quai is beleieved to stop hair loss and even regrow hair.

3. Saw Palmetto – A small creeping palm – Also known as Serenoa repens. It contains free fatty acids and phytosterols, which block the formation of DHT and by inhibiting the enzyme 5-alpha reductase that contributes to androgenetic alopecia and has been shown to be more effective than Finasteride in some cases.

4. Aloe Vera – Taken from the inner leaves of plants, it is a substance in a gel formation that is known for its ability to calm irritated skin. It protects the scalp and hair and also known as a good remedy against Alopecia.

5. Capsicum – A type of hot peppers which stimulates hair growth by at least half and increases blood flow to the scalp. This herb is good for regrowing hair.

6. Lemongrass – A pale green stalk about 18 inches long. This herb stables oil product in the scalp. It also increases fullness and body to the hair.

If you suffer from hair loss or thinning hair or just want to keep your hair healthy and strong, it is recommended to use herbal hair loss treatments.

Super Power – Antioxidants for Your Hair

Antioxidants are power nutrients that help our overall health as well as are protective of hair. Free radicals are unstable atoms within the body. These radicals work havoc on healthy cells. They have been linked to such diseases as Alzheimer's, cancer, arthritis and many inflammatory conditions within the body.

The purpose of antioxidants is to help protect the cells from the free radicals. Antioxidants stop the oxidizing effects of free radicals. A perfect example would be what happens when we eat an apple. After you eat an apple if you leave it exposed to the air (oxygen) it will begin to turn brown. That process is called oxidation. However if you take that same apple and squeeze lemon juice over it, the oxidation will slow down. It is the Vitamin C in the lemon that counteracts the oxidizing effect of free radicals.

The most powerful antioxidants are Vitamin A, C and E. It is advantageous to take antioxidant supplements and eat a diet high in antioxidants. Here is a list of foods that contain high levels of antioxidants. Help yourself to these nutrient dense foods.

Super Power Foods

Oranges

Lemons

Limes

Grapes

Cherries

Pineapple

Pears

Cantaloupe

Strawberries

Raspberries

Plums

Carrots

Tomatoes

Green peppers

Mushrooms

Beans

Broccoli

Onions

Cabbage

Sweet potatoes

Squash

Collard greens

Mustard greens

Turnip greens

Potatoes

Wheat Germ

Soy Beans

Nuts

Sunflower seeds

Liver

Eggs

Milk

Whole grains

Whole grain breads

Whole grain cereal

Suggested value for antioxidant supplements:

A – This is not a water-soluble vitamin so check with your health care practitioner.

C – Minimum of 60 mg.

E – Up to 400 IU

Soothing Treatments for Your Hair

Your scalp loves to be pampered. Did you know that there are common thing that you already have in your home that your hair and scalp would love? Did you know that there are inexpensive items that you can buy at the grocery store that will greatly benefit your hair and scalp? We would like to share a few of these with you.

Common home products

Mayonnaise is a great product that can be used to condition the hair.

Honey mixed with olive oil (or other essential oil) plus cinnamon powder can be rubbed into the scalp for 15 minutes. This is a growth treatment.

Apple Cider Vinegar and water can help to clean and detoxify the scalp.

Coconut oil is great for moisturizing the hair.

Inexpensive store products

Aloe Vera gel used once a week to wash your hair.

Coconut milk and green coconut can be applied to the hair. Leave it on for and hour and a half.

Henna has been used traditionally for hair growth.

Soothing Through Aromatherapy for Your Hair

Our ancestors did not have the benefit of today's scientifically researched drugs, but they often found natural remedies that worked just as well. Herbal remedies have been used for centuries to treat everything from premenstrual syndrome to high blood pressure. Men experiencing the first signs of baldness often looked to natural cures as well, and some of the herbal remedies have surprising results.

A group of dermatologists in Scotland tested an herbal remedy with great success, helping over 40% of their patients with a mixture of essential oils containing cedarwood, lavender, rosemary and thyme. In this double blind study, the group using the essential oils showed improvement in 40 percent of the subjects, while only 15% of the control group noted an improvement.

So, would you be interested in trying out aromatherapy as a hair loss solution? If you'd like to experiment with this, mix three drops each of lavender and rosemary oil with two drops each of cedarwood and thyme oils. Add this mixture to 4 teaspoons of grapeseed oil and one-quarter teaspoon of jojoba oil. Rub the mixture into your scalp for two minutes nightly, and then use a warm towel to wrap your head.

If you're not experiencing baldness yet, but your hair doesn't

look healthy, you may want to try a mixture of lavender and

bay essential oils to stimulate blood flow to the scalp and help

circulation to the area. About six drops of oil, each, should be

added.

Section Two

Natural Hair Care

Natural Hair Care

As encouraged from earlier in this book it is essential that you be very proactive in uncovering the root cause of your hair loss problem. But this should be an on going process. Always be on the take to finding things that can specifically improve your condition. Hair loss solutions for one person may not be the hair loss solution that works for you, but you can gain insight and knowledge into the scope of hair loss complexities. Continue studying until you find the resources that specifically work for you.

We know the most common conditions associated with hair loss:

Genetics

Hormonal imbalance

Improper hair care

Health issues

Diet

We know what is necessary to begin the journey for hair care recovery:

Understanding how hair grows - Anagen, Catagen and Telogen phases

Understanding the types of hair loss

Understanding how stress affects hair loss

Understanding hair care from a cellular level

Understanding hair care from an herbal level

Understanding hair care through the power of antioxidants

Understanding hair care through soothing treatments to calm the scalp

Understanding hair care through aromatherapy

In this section we're going to learn about natural hair care. As long as there are live hair follicles on your scalp and no scaring tissues, your chances of recovery are greater; even if it's related to genetics or Androgen imbalances. For recovery, it is highly recommended that you stop all chemical treatments to your hair – relaxers, coloring, etc. and allow your hair natural state to emerge.

Hair Recovery

Here are some tips that will help your hair to recover. Understand the importance of massaging the scalp. Massaging the scalp increases blow flow. Increased circulation aids in recovery. It is also suggested that as you massage the scalp to add hair oil to your process. Two of the best oils for your hair are olive oil and castor oil.

Here are some of the benefits for olive oil for your scalp.

High in antioxidants

Anti inflammatory

Anti bacterial

Here are some of the benefits to using castor oil for your scalp:

Anti bacterial

Excellent source of Vitamin E

Mineral rich

High in Omega 6 and 9 Fatty Acids

Massaging your scalp with these oils and adding wheat sprout can greatly help your recovery. Try rotating the oils and wheat sprout every two days. To increase the benefits put a hot towel on your head for about thirty minutes after the massage.

The ultimate to increase blow flow is to do head stands. We will not suggest that you stand on your head, but we do want to educate you that process is available. Blood will go directly to the scalp and provide nutrients to the hair follicle. You may want to consider a modified motion by bending over placing your head to its lowest level for a few minutes.

Another helpful tip is to become more aware of the foods that can help your hair to recover. Biotin is one of those nutrients that can help. Here are a list of some biotin rich foods:

Green peas

Nuts

Brown rice

Seeds

Walnuts

Egg yolks

Sweet potatoes

Food yeast

Mushrooms

Carrots

Cauliflower

Salmon

Avocadoes

Whole grains

Spinach

Besides biotin, one of the other best nutrient dense products to us is zinc. Zinc helps to restore damage to cells and it strengthen your body tissue. Keeping your iron levels maximized is also very important because oxygen in supplied to the body through iron. Hair follicles needed to be oxygenated. Lucerne is another word for Alfalfa, is also important to hair recovery. It has the capacity to strength your hair and to reduce your chances of hair loss. It contains high levels of B1 and B6 that are beneficial to your hair, and it is rich in minerals. It comes in powder form and can be easily added to any beverage of your choice.

Reasons for Choosing Natural Hair Products

Hair care products are a huge and unregulated industry. Yes, unregulated. The U.S. Food and Drug Administration classify the products but don't have any regulating standards for what goes into those bottles. You may be shocked to find out what your body ingests with the hair care products use. Even those listed as "all natural" may have synthetic bi products and emulsifiers. While you are thinking that you are optimizing your hair products, you may have bought into the industry game. Therefore it is important to read the label and know what is being used. The more that you are able to identify a product without having to look it up is a tip that the product truly is all-natural. For example if it says rosemary oil, you know that is all natural. But if it says sodium lauryl sulfate you would have to look that up to determine if it were natural or not.

The list below will provide common products used in shampoos that you might want to become very aware of, as these contents do impact the health of your hair.

Synthetic fragrances

Problems caused – rashes, headaches, vomiting and dizziness

Diethanolamine

Problems caused in lab rats – cancer and toxic to the brain

Propylene Glycol

Problems caused – allergic conditions

Sodium lauryl sulfate

Problem caused – asthma trigger, hair follicle damage

Ammonium lauryl

Problem caused – eye irritation, hair follicle damage

Having this understanding of the need to identify the type of products that you are using on your body will aide to you making better choices concerning your hair care. We would again suggest, using the most natural products for your hair at all times. That particular choice will give your hair the greatest chance of recovery.

Natural Hair Choices

On the whole, our society is becoming much more in tune with the need to start living more naturally, pure lives. People are starting to pay attention to the ways in which their favorite items have been made and the ingredients that have been used. This is a great start, but there are even more options out there for people to discover.

The items that we use to make ourselves fresh and beautiful can actually contain harsh synthetic ingredients that can have the exact opposite effect. People who are not using natural hair care products need to learn about the benefits that these items can have.

By entering the shower and reaching for a naturally produced item, everyone can enjoy the benefits that purity offers. Pure ingredients are sourced from beautiful and exotic places such as the Amazon rainforest or the grasslands of Africa. Imagine linking yourself to these fascinating places with every shampoo and conditioner.

Everyone wants to look their very best, but some items create better effects than others. Some companies produce inexpensive, low-quality products that are heavily laden with chemicals and then sell them to us at a high cost. Unlike natural hair care products, chemically based ones can sometimes strip the beauty from hair.

Naturally produced items contain only the purest ingredients to ensure that they provide a deep cleansing without leaving a filmy residue. These items create a soft and light lather that provides moisture and shine. Using only the finest ingredients such as essential oils means that these items make your mane look its very best.

Natural hair care products are designed to provide the lift and sheen that everyone looks for. The secret to achieving the best locks possible is to provide your hair with all the right vitamins and nutrients that it requires. Naturally produced treatments are able to give the right balance without the use of harsh chemicals.

Everyone knows that using the perfect product is a matter of knowing about the needs of their unique hair. Some people's locks are limp and lifeless, other people suffer from too much oil, and still others have the dried and frizzy looks. Naturally produced items provide the range of treatments that can suit everyone and their special needs.

In addition, with natural hair care products there is a lot less risk of over processing. You are unlikely to find that your mane becomes dry or split after using a naturally produced item. Similarly, items that contain only the purest ingredients will not cause dry scalp or greasy roots.

African American Hair Texture and Care

African American hair is diverse in texture ranging from super tight and coily to thick and loose curls. Whatever the texture is, it reflects our varied ethnic diversity in that our race in genetically unique, a blend of many cultures through predominantly African. It is truly a gift to have our hair texture, but we often don't feel that way because we are at war with our hair both personally and socially. It is only recently that African Americans have come to accept their hair as it is upon their heads, and not care what others think. This is a great revelatory understanding.

Understanding The Basics

One of the first thing that African American women must do is to decide if they are willing to go through life with their natural hair or permed hair. There are pros and cons associated with each methodology. However in order to determine how to care for your hair, the choice has to be made.

The next basic is to understand that taking care of your hair starts from the inside out. Therefore make sure to eat a diet that gives you all of the nutrients that your hair needs to grow. It also means making sure to keep yourself hydrated. Water really does contribute to hair growth. So make sure that you have an adequate intake of water to keep your body and hair moisturized.

The Proper Comb/Brush

What type of comb/brush do you use on your hair? Regardless of your hair texture it is really important to have a proper comb/brush. Make sure to use one that fits your ethnicity. African American women need to use a comb/brush that is wide and easily can comb through their hair. Most combs on the market are made for straight hair. Be smart and really observe what you are using. If it is not wide enough to fit through the curly tresses of African American hair then it should not be used. A broad comb/brush will act to detangle the hair and will help to prevent breakage. That is critical for the health of African American hair.

Other Steps

Once you have established the proper comb/brush routine there are other things that will help you to maintain your hair. Make sure that you use heat in small amounts. If your hair is permed using heat can be harmful so try using the lowest heat setting that will thoroughly dry your hair. Next make sure that you are not washing your hair too often. Washing African American hair every seven to ten days can really help keep the hair healthy. Always get in the habit of using a daily leave in conditioner. Treat yourself to a lavish deep conditioning once a month.

Love Your Texture

Learn to love your hair. Understand that African American hair is unique to our culture and should be enjoyed. Find a way to manage your hair type and enjoy it. Don't look at what others do to their hair. Find your own unique pathway. Embrace the fact that every hair care product will not work with your particular texture, and find the ones that will. This will insure that not only is your hair getting the best treatment, but will help you to enjoy your hair as you see how it responds to the right type of hair care. The result is that you will feel more beautiful and reflect that confidence to the world. Embrace the fact that diversity makes the world a beautiful place and that you are a part of the beauty.

The last tip that we will share for African American women is to find a hair salon that will work for you. Don't be afraid to try different places until you have the right professionals that can work with your unique hair texture.

Conclusion

I hope that you have enjoyed reading Hair Loss Solutions. We hope that we have provided you with an understanding of the conditions surrounding hair loss, provided solutions, and introduced you to the best way to begin your journey – with a hair loss team. Most of all we hope that we have given you encouragement that you can recover from hair loss.

If we can assist you with your hair loss journey please contact Leola Anifowhoshe, Chief Trichologist at:

Solutions Hair Restoration Center

3727 Greenbriar Dr. #109 B

Stafford, TX 77469

Office 832 886-4653

https://solutionshairrestoration.weebly.com/

www.ingramcontent.com/pod-product-compliance
Lightning Source LLC
Chambersburg PA
CBHW061732250726

48657CB00002B/889